UNDERSTANDING ARTHRITIS

DR DECLAN HARVEY

Table of Contents

Chapter One

Introduction

Arthritis refers to a group of diseases that cause inflammation and stiffness in the joints. This can lead to pain, reduced range of motion, and difficulty with daily activities.

The exact cause of most types of arthritis is still unknown. However, researchers have identified various risk factors that can contribute to the development of arthritis, including:

- Age: As people get older, the risk of developing arthritis increases.
- Genetics: Some forms of arthritis, such as rheumatoid arthritis, can run in families.
- Gender: Women are more likely to develop rheumatoid arthritis, while men are more susceptible to gout.
- Obesity: Being overweight puts extra stress on the joints, leading to an increased risk of arthritis.

- Joint injuries: A history of joint injuries or overuse can increase the likelihood of developing osteoarthritis.
- Infections: Certain infections can trigger the development of reactive arthritis, which causes inflammation in the joints.
- Autoimmune disorders: Conditions like lupus or psoriasis can increase the risk of developing certain types of arthritis.

- Smoking: Smoking has been linked to an increased risk of rheumatoid arthritis.

- In addition to these risk factors, there may also be a combination of environmental, genetic, and hormonal factors that contribute to the development of arthritis. It is essential to consult with a healthcare professional for an accurate diagnosis and personalized treatment plan for arthritis.

Types Of Arthritis

There are over 100 different types of arthritis, but the most common types include:

- Osteoarthritis: This is the most common form of arthritis, caused by wear and tear of the joints, often seen in older adults.

- Rheumatoid arthritis: This is an autoimmune disorder in which the body's immune system attacks the joints, causing inflammation and damage.

- Psoriatic arthritis: This type of arthritis is associated with the skin condition psoriasis, and can cause joint pain, stiffness, and swelling.
- Gout: This is a form of arthritis caused by the buildup of uric acid crystals in the joints, leading to sudden, severe pain.
- Juvenile arthritis: This refers to various types of arthritis that develop in

children under the age of
16.

- Ankylosing spondylitis: This is a type of inflammatory arthritis that primarily affects the spine and can lead to loss of mobility.
- Reactive arthritis: This type of arthritis is caused by an infection in another part of the body, typically the urinary tract or gastrointestinal tract.
- Systemic lupus erythematosus: This is an autoimmune disorder

that can cause joint pain and damage, along with a range of other symptoms.

- Fibromyalgia: This is a chronic condition that causes widespread muscle pain and tenderness, and can also affect the joints.
- Osteoporosis: While not technically a type of arthritis, osteoporosis is a common condition in which bones become weak and brittle, often leading to fractures.

Understanding Arthritis

Anatomy Of Joints

According to findings presented by the Johns Hopkins Medicine group, almost 1 in 4 adults in the United States have been diagnosed with some form of arthritis. This makes arthritis a common, yet often misunderstood condition. Before discussing the specific anatomy of joints affected by arthritis, it is important to understand what arthritis is and what causes it.

Arthritis is a broad term that refers to inflammation of the joints. There are over 100 different types of arthritis that can affect different joints in the body. The two most common forms of arthritis are osteoarthritis and rheumatoid arthritis.

Osteoarthritis is caused by wear and tear on the joints over time, while rheumatoid arthritis is an autoimmune disorder where the body's immune system attacks the joints. Both types of arthritis can cause pain, stiffness, and swelling in the joints, limiting movement and affecting daily activities.

Now, let's take a closer look at the anatomy of joints affected by arthritis.

- Cartilage : Cartilage is a connective tissue found in our joints that provides a smooth surface for bones to glide over each other. In healthy joints, cartilage acts as a shock absorber, cushioning the bones and protecting them from damage during movement. In arthritic joints, the cartilage breaks down or wears away, leaving the bones in the joint exposed and without protection.

- Synovium : The synovium is a thin, flexible lining that surrounds the joint. It produces synovial fluid, which lubricates the joint and helps reduce friction between the bones. In arthritis, the synovium becomes inflamed, leading to a buildup of excess fluid in the joint, causing pain and stiffness.

- Ligaments : Ligaments are strong bands of tissue that connect bones to each other and provide stability to the joint. In arthritis, these ligaments can become stretched or damaged, leading to instability and weakness of the joint.
- Bones: Bones are the hard, mineralized

structures that make up our skeleton. In joints affected by arthritis, the bones may become damaged or deformed due to the breakdown of cartilage and changes in the surrounding tissues, leading to pain and limited mobility.

- Muscles and Tendons: Muscles and tendons work together to move the joints, with the tendons connecting muscles to bones. In arthritis, the muscles surrounding the affected joint may become weak or atrophied due to decreased use and pain, while the tendons can become inflamed or torn, causing further discomfort and limited range of motion.

Physiology of inflammation

Inflammation is a normal physiological response of the immune system to injury, infection, or irritation. It is an important part of the body's defense mechanism and helps to protect against harmful substances and to promote healing. When the body detects an irritant or damage to its cells, it triggers a complex chain of events to fight off the threat and repair any damage. This response involves the recruitment of immune cells, release of inflammatory molecules, and increased blood flow to the affected area.

The process of inflammation is controlled by a network of chemicals and cells, including cytokines, chemokines, and immune cells such as white blood cells. These substances work together to identify and neutralize the irritant, remove damaged cells and tissues, and promote healing.

Inflammation can be categorized as either acute or chronic. Acute inflammation is a short-term response that is triggered by a specific injury or infection and is characterized by swelling, redness, pain, and heat. This type of inflammation is essential for the body to heal and typically resolves within a few days or weeks. Chronic inflammation, on the other hand, is a prolonged response that can last for months or even years. It may be caused by persistent irritants such as toxins, pathogens, or autoimmune reactions. Chronic inflammation can damage healthy tissues and can lead to various diseases, including arthritis.

In the case of arthritis, chronic inflammation occurs in

the joints, leading to pain, stiffness, and loss of function. The immune system attacks the lining of the joint, called the synovium, causing it to become inflamed and swollen. This inflammation can also damage cartilage and bone within the joint, leading to further pain and stiffness.

Inflammatory arthritis is a type of arthritis that is caused by an overactive immune system, resulting in chronic inflammation in the joints. Examples of inflammatory arthritis include rheumatoid arthritis, psoriatic arthritis, and ankylosing spondylitis.

In addition to causing joint pain and damage, chronic inflammation can also have systemic effects on the body. It has been linked to cardiovascular disease, diabetes, and other chronic conditions. Therefore, managing inflammation is an important aspect of addressing arthritis and its associated health effects.

How Arthritis Affects The Body

Arthritis is a joint disorder that causes inflammation, stiffness, and pain in one or more joints in the body. There are over 100 different types of arthritis, but the most common types are osteoarthritis and rheumatoid arthritis.

- Cartilage damage : One of the main effects of arthritis on the body is damage to the cartilage that covers the ends of bones in a joint. Cartilage is a firm, rubbery tissue that cushions the bones and allows them to glide smoothly against each other. In arthritis, the cartilage gradually breaks down, leading to bone-on-bone contact and causing pain and stiffness.

- Inflammation: Inflammation is a natural response of the body's immune system to injury or infection. In arthritis, the inflammation is chronic, meaning it is ongoing and long-lasting. This inflammation causes the tissues in and around the joint to become swollen, stiff, and painful.

- Joint stiffness and pain : Inflammation and cartilage damage both lead to joint stiffness and pain, which are common symptoms of arthritis. The pain may be constant or come and go and can range from mild to severe. The stiffness often makes it difficult to move the affected joint, and in some cases, the joint may become completely immobile.

- Joint deformities : In some forms of arthritis, such as rheumatoid arthritis, the inflammation may cause the joint to become deformed over time. As the disease progresses, the cartilage and bone in the joint may erode, leading to visible changes in the joint's shape and structure.

- Limited range of motion : As arthritis causes inflammation, stiffness, and pain in the affected joint, it can also limit the joint's range of motion. This means that the joint may not be able to move as freely as before, making it difficult to perform daily activities like walking, climbing stairs, or holding objects.
- Soft tissue damage : The inflamed tissue in and

around the joint may also cause damage to the surrounding ligaments, tendons, and muscles. This can lead to weakness and instability in the joint, making it more prone to injury.

- Fatigue: Arthritis can cause fatigue, which is a feeling of extreme tiredness and lack of energy. This is due to the body's constant fight against the inflammation in the joints, which can drain the body's energy reserves.

- **Loss of function and disability** : As arthritis progresses, it can cause significant damage to the joints and surrounding tissues, leading to loss of function and disability. This can greatly impact a person's ability to perform daily tasks and lead to a decreased quality of life.

In addition to these physical effects, arthritis can also have a significant emotional and psychological impact on a person, causing stress, anxiety, and depression. It is important to seek medical treatment and support to manage the symptoms and impact of arthritis on the body.

Signs And Symptoms Of Arthritis

- Joint pain: This is the most common sign of arthritis. The pain may be dull, sharp, or burning and may occur at rest or when moving the affected joint.

- Stiffness: Arthritis can cause stiffness in the affected joints, making movement difficult and painful.
- Swelling: Inflammation of the joint can cause swelling, which can be seen and felt.
- Redness and warmth: The affected joint may appear red and feel warm to the touch due to increased blood flow and inflammation.

- Difficulty moving: As arthritis progresses, it can limit the range of motion in the affected joint, making it difficult to perform everyday tasks.
- Fatigue: Arthritis can cause fatigue and a feeling of being unwell, especially during a flare-up.
- Loss of flexibility: With ongoing inflammation and stiffness, the affected joint may lose

its flexibility, making it difficult to move.

- Muscle weakness: Weakness in the muscles surrounding the affected joint may occur due to lack of use or pain.
- Joint clicking or popping: As the cartilage in the joint wears away, it may cause a clicking or popping sound when moving the joint.
- Deformity: In some forms of arthritis, such as rheumatoid arthritis, joints may become

deformed and appear misaligned.

- Numbness and tingling: Arthritis can sometimes cause nerve compression, leading to numbness, tingling, or burning sensations in the affected area.
- Fever: Some types of arthritis, such as rheumatoid arthritis, can cause fever and flu-like symptoms during flare-ups.
- Loss of appetite: Arthritis can cause a loss of

appetite and weight loss, especially during periods of active inflammation.

- Insomnia: Chronic pain and discomfort can make it difficult to sleep, leading to insomnia and fatigue.

- Mood changes: Dealing with chronic pain and limited mobility can lead to mood changes, such as anxiety, depression, and irritability.

Diagnostic Procedures Of Arthritis

- Physical Examination: This involves a thorough assessment of the joints and surrounding structures, looking for any signs of swelling, tenderness, warmth, or deformity. The doctor may also evaluate joint range of motion and muscle strength.
- X-ray: This imaging test uses low levels of radiation to produce

detailed pictures of bones and joints. It can help detect joint changes such as narrowing of joint space, bone spurs, and loss of cartilage.

- Magnetic Resonance Imaging (MRI): This imaging test uses a magnetic field and radio waves to create detailed images of bones, soft tissues, and organs. It can help identify inflammation, damage to tendons and ligaments, and other soft tissue abnormalities.

- Ultrasound: This imaging technique uses high-frequency sound waves to produce images of soft tissues and structures within the body. It can help detect joint inflammation, fluid accumulation, and other abnormalities.

- Blood Tests: These tests can help identify markers of inflammation, such as levels of C-reactive protein (CRP) and erythrocyte sedimentation rate (ESR). Blood tests can also be used to detect specific antibodies that are associated with different types of arthritis.

- Joint Aspiration: This procedure involves using a needle and syringe to remove fluid from an inflamed joint. The fluid can be analyzed for signs of infection, inflammation, or other causes.

- Synovial Biopsy: In this procedure, a small sample of tissue is taken from the lining of an affected joint and examined under a microscope. It can help diagnose the type of arthritis and determine the severity of the condition.

- Arthroscopy: This is a minimally invasive procedure where a small camera is inserted into the joint through a small incision. This allows the doctor to visually examine the joint and take tissue samples if needed.

- Electromyography (EMG): This is a test that evaluates the electrical activity of muscles. It can help distinguish between arthritis and other conditions, such as nerve compression or muscle disorders.
- Nerve Conduction Studies: This test measures how well electrical impulses travel

through nerves. It can help diagnose nerve damage or compression, which can cause symptoms similar to arthritis.

THE END

www.ingramcontent.com/pod-product-compliance
Lightning Source LLC
Chambersburg PA
CBHW071553260726
48653CB00008BA/3074